WILL-POWER AND ITS DEVELOPMENT

Swami Budhananda

Advaita Ashrama
(PUBLICATION DEPARTMENT)
5 DEHI ENTALLY ROAD · KOLKATA 700 014

Published by
Swami Bodhasarananda
Adhyaksha, Advaita Ashrama
Mayavati, Champawat, Uttarakhand
from its Publication Department, Kolkata
Email: mail@advaitaashrama.org
Website: www.advaitaashrama.org

© *All Rights Reserved*
First Edition, 1990
Thirtieth Impression, March 2009
20M6C

ISBN 978-81-85301-64-8

Printed in India at
Trio Process
Kolkata 700 014

PUBLISHER'S NOTE

Will-power and Its Development by Swami Budhananda first appeared in the May and June issues of the *Prabuddha Bharata* of 1983. Many of our readers who were impressed by the importance of the subject matter and the quality of the article requested us time and again to publish it in the form of a brochure for the benefit of a wider public. We are therefore bringing out this small booklet with the hope that it will help to develop in them an indomitable will-power which is a *sine qua non* for success in the life of every human being.

Swami Budhananda, an erudite scholar and a forceful writer, was for some years the Editor of the *Prabuddha Bharata* and President of the Advaita Ashrama, Mayavati and passed away in 1983.

1 January 1990   PUBLISHER

CONTENTS

1. Twofold ideal of life 7
2. Will-power : the secret of success 8
3. How the will originates 11
4. The cause of small and big tragedies of life 13
5. How to generate will-power in the human system 21
6. Remedies for failure of will-power ... 37
7. Caution needed for properly directing will-power 40
8. Behold the triumph of will-power ... 42
9. The great option open to all 47

WILL-POWER AND ITS DEVELOPMENT

Twofold ideal of life

Indian religious tradition teaches that human beings, generally speaking, can have two commendable aspirations. One is called *abhyudaya* or worldly prosperity and well-being; the other is called *niḥśreyasa* or spiritual illumination and freedom. Of these both *dharma* or righteousness is said to be the basis. Prosperity that has not *dharma* as the basis crumbles down sooner than feared due to internal haemorrhage, so to say. Of course, spiritual illumination one cannot even think of except through being righteous.

Further it is taught, that if *abhyudaya* or worldly prosperity is not directed and subordinated to, and utilized for, attaining *niḥśreyasa*, spiritual illumination, it becomes self-destructive. We must however, clearly understand that from prosperity illumination is not a logical development, though 'empty stomach is no good for religion'.

Will-power: the secret of success

Now, this one thing we all definitely want in life: success. Whatever may be our undertakings—in the direction of worldly prosperity or spiritual illumination, in spheres secular or spiritual—not one of us likes to fail. We all want to succeed. Success though we all desire, it will be noticed in various spheres of life, truly successful men are only a handful. Many are those who attain only a moderate degree of success. And many more just fail.

There will be various factors in the stories of men's successes and failures of life. But in every single case there will be one common factor involved. That is the factor of will-power. The degree of a person's success in life is commensurate with the degree of will-power he has attained.

'How to develop the will-power' thus turns out to be the most important fundamental issue of everyone's life. It should be the part of our education from our childhood to be trained in developing the will-power, for without it education remains largely ineffective. Swami Vivekananda says:

> What is education? Is it book-learning? No. Is it diverse knowledge? Not even that. The training by which the current and expression of will are brought under control and become fruitful is called education. Now consider, is that education as a result of which the will, being continuously choked by force through generations, is now well-nigh killed out; is that education under whose sway even the old ideas, let alone new ones, are disappearing one by one; is that education which is slowly making man a machine?[1]

If, unfortunately, we have not learnt how to develop will-power early in life, we should do so at any stage of life, because self-improvement is almost impossible without the voluntary or involuntary exercise

---

1 *The Complete Works of Swami Vivekananda* (Calcutta : Advaita Ashrama, 1988), vol. 4, p. 490.

of the will-power. Whereas, given the will-power, we can bring about considerable changes in our individual and also collective lives for the better, from very hopeless situations.

Consider these three cases of modern history. When Lincoln was alone with history in the White House in those dark days of Civil War, what would have happened to the Union but for his powerful will to save it? Consider how the will-power of Winston Churchill played the decisive role in the 2nd World War. What would have happened to England and Europe now enjoying prosperity but for that man's will who said he had nothing else to offer but blood, sweat and tears? Consider again the effect of the will-power of Gandhiji, whom Churchill called 'the half-naked fakir', for all the poeples in the world who in their own lands were ruled by colonial powers?

If we study the lives of those persons who were once in very bad shape and afterwards were found to rise from the shambles in a spectacular manner, we shall discover, in every single case, it was their will-power that brought about their transformation and rise. If we study the lives of some persons who early in life showed much promise, had enviable facility to rise high, and yet never fulfilled their promise, wilting away like buds before fully blossoming, we shall discover in every single case that there it was the absence of the will-power that caused their early wilting.

Given the will-power, man makes everything out of nothing as it were. In the absence of the will-power, all his talents and qualities and endowments come to nothing.

How the will originates

In the Vedas it is said:

> This universe, in truth, in the beginning was nothing at all. There was no heaven, no earth, no atmosphere. This being, that was solely non-being, conceived a wish: 'May I be.'[2]

Whether you accept or reject the content of this cosmogony, one truth comes out of it: that behind all creative efforts in all spheres of life is an act of will. But what is will? Wherefrom does it originate? 'Will is a compound of the self and mind,'[3] says Swami

---

2 *Taittirīya Brāhmaṇa*, 2.2.9.1.
3 *Complete Works* (1972), vol. 6, p. 44.

Vivekananda. By the word 'self' is meant here the Atman or the real soul of man. Atman is beyond causation. It is undifferentiated consciousness. In that consciousness there is no will, because will presupposes reaction to something external or other. In undifferentiated consciousness there is no such thing. Though Atman is free in its pure essential nature, when identified with mind and body, it is in a state of bondage. In other words, in that state Atman is not free. The will is the first manifestation of the real self caught in phenomena or maya. It is a compound of Atman and mind, and mind is subtle matter. Therefore in the will there are two strands: one of the spirit and the other of matter—a strand of light and a strand of darkness.

In the ultimate analysis, however, this compound is bound to be unreal, for it is based on the unreality of maya. But as long as we are in the realm of maya, that is to say, as long as we remain spiritually unillumined it is very real for all practical purposes. And it moves things in the way which nothing else does in the world, except the powerful forces of nature.

Even these great forces are surmounted by the force of human will. Imagine what was the face of America in the days of Columbus, or even what the Pilgrim Fathers saw, and compare it with the face of America today. These vast and stupendous changes were all brought about by human will. All the actions we see in the world, all the movements and achievements of man are manifestations of the will of man. What we are proud of, and what we deplore in human civilization; what amazes us in the spheres of science, and what makes us speechless in the domain of religion, are all manifestations of the will of man. As Swami Vivekananda says, 'This will is caused by character and character is manufactured by Karma or work. As is the Karma so is the manifestation of the will.'[4]

The cause of small and big tragedies of life

Let us now understand this concept of will-power from a practical point of view as it affects our life. Why at all need we develop the will-power when we may not be ambitious people trying to do spectacular things? Sometimes in our lives, maybe in every one's

---

4 *Complete Works* (1972), vol. 1, p. 30.

life, great tragedies happen. They shake us to our roots. After that tragedy we are never the same persons again. If we know how to take these tragedies creatively, we are largely transformed. If not, we are crushed. These tragedies are such that we are forced to take agonizing notice of them. Not only that, others also take notice of them, for very often we become objects of real pity. This is about the big tragedies of our personal lives.

There is another kind of tragedy which is daily happening in every life, the consequences of which are far-reaching. And in these small tragedies are rooted the great tragedies of life. But, somehow, most people seem not to notice them at all. These days, we are giving away our thinking power to machines in the hope of getting more out of life. But it would appear, by and large, we are gradually losing grip on life. It may not be an axiomatic truth, but we shall find it to be generally true that the more our homes become filled with gadgets, the less are the thoughtful people around.

The one way of keeping grip on life is right thinking and deep thinking. These days we all admire free-thinking. Free-thinking is good. But right thinking is better. When right

WILL-POWER AND ITS DEVELOPMENT

thinking becomes deep thinking, it is excellent. Without cultivating the habit of introspection, it is impossible to keep track of all the forces that are operative within us. Without knowing the nature of these forces, we cannot be their masters. We are then bound to be their slaves. And what chances have slaves to develop and exercise their will-power, when that slavery is due to their own unregenerate nature? How can such persons ever build up their character? How can a man without a character have will-power?

Introspection will reveal that there is a basic tragedy involved in our daily life, in which most of our big tragedies are rooted. In Sanskrit this basic tragedy is narrated this way: 'I know what is *dharma*, what is righteousness, what is good, but I have not the inclination to do it. I know what is unrighteousness, *adharma*, what is evil, sin, but I cannot desist from doing it.'[5] A song of the mystic Ramprasad, which Sri Ramakrishna used to sing piteously describes the content of

---

5 जानामि धर्म न च मे प्रवृत्तिः ।
जानाम्यधर्म न च मे निवृत्तिः ।।

Prapanna Gītā (or *Pāṇḍava Gītā*)

this tragedy:

> O Mother, I have none else to blame;
> Alas! I sink in the well these very hands
>   have dug,
> With the six passions for my spade,
> I dug a pit in the sacred land of earth;
> And now the dark water of death
>   gushes forth!
> How can I save myself, O my Redeemer?
> Surely I have been my own enemy;
> How can I now ward off this
>   dark water of death?
> Behold, the waters rise to my chest!
> How can I save myself? O Mother,
>   save me!
> Thou art my only Refuge;
>   with Thy protecting glance,
> Take me across to the other shore of the
> world.[6]

In its fullness the basic tragedy of our daily life leads to such spiritual crisis, about which Ramprasad laments before the Divine Mother.

---

[6] Translation of Ramprasad's song quoted from 'M' *The Gospel of Sri Ramakrishna* (Madras : Sri Ramakrishna Math, 1981), p. 203.

So then, the basic tragedy of our life is: (a) our inability to do the thing we know to be right and helpful; as well as, (b) our incapacity to desist from doing what we know to be wrong, unhelpful, if not disastrous.

We know it is good to use polite, decent and restrained language, in our daily dealings at home, on the street, in business, in politics, in society. But, in spite of ourselves, we use wrong language, from which arise many dissensions, small and big, at home, in society, in national and international affairs. Very often we do not remember the power of words, their capacity to break or make, wound or heal. More often, our will just fails to carry into practice what we know about the power of words. Through use of wrong language we are apt to make such wounds in others' hearts as will not be easily healed; or we may anger people to such an extent that dire consequences may follow. And we ourselves shall have to reap them, however bitter they may be.

We know that it is beneficial to live a moral life, yet, in spite of ourselves, we commit sinful acts. And having committed them we have to take their painful consequences. We can give away our entire property but there is no way of giving away the fruits of our karma. We shall have to enjoy or suffer them ourselves. We know it is good to live according to the commandments of religion and obey the precepts of the Guru. We know it is good to get up early in the morning and practise spiritual disciplines. But when in the morning the alarm clock dutifully rings, we feel annoyed and silence it as though it had committed some crime, and then pull the blanket over the nose and sleep half an hour more, only to hurry and worry all day long. In the evening when we return home we are a mass of tension, and so highly inflammable that any little thing is apt to set things on fire.

We may observe, even in little things how little of what we know to be good for us, to be beneficial for us, we are able to put into practice. On the contrary, we continue to do harmful things. We know it is not good to neglect our studies, but somehow we cannot turn our ears or eyes from the radio or TV, specially when a cricket match, a circus show, a fashion show or a movie is going on. If our mind timidly protests, we just give it a thrashing: how can I miss such an exciting thing, for the boring bla-bla-bla of my classes? And the consequences of it are too obvious in the ever growing restlessness and dissatisfaction among the youngsters.

Do not people very well know that it is not good to drink alcohol? Still they gulp one or two glasses first occasionally, then more, compulsively. They promise not to drink only to break the promise again. Ultimately they even fail to promise. I believe it was Will Rogers who said: 'Well, it is quite easy to give up smoking. I have done it a hundred times!' But the record of Alcoholic Anonymous shows it is possible to start a new life as it were, by developing a new will to live a different kind of life.

We know that over-weight is a health hazard, and we should avoid eating too many sweets and other highly fattening things. But when these things come round, we smile away our own mental decisions and opposition of well-wishers.

It is well-known that some of us can resist everything except temptations! There is a great fascination in the prohibited, great attraction in the destructive, great pull in the bizarre and wicked things in this world of maya. They pull us by the ear and make slaves of us. We do things in a hurry and then repent at leisure, and weep in the darkness of our own making.

Now, why do we behave this way knowingly? We do wrong things unknowingly too. But, that apart, why do we do wrong things and fail to do right things, knowingly? We must not commit the mistake of thinking that we do such things because we are essentially wicked or because of some kind of 'original sin' in us or because of our being forced by evil powers. Let us know it for certain that no one in this world is essentially wicked. Essentially everyone is divine, because the essence of every being is Atman, which is divine. The apparent wickedness of any person is only a fortuity, an outer mask, and hence it can be gotten rid of. No cow tells a lie. A tree does not steal or rob. A stone slab does not commit burglary. Only man does all these. But a cow, as far as we know, cannot think of God. A tree cannot practise spiritual disciplines. A stone slab cannot realize God. But man can.

The inescapable conclusion, then, is that the basic daily tragedies of our lives are not rooted in any inalienable, essential wickedness in us, but in the failure of our will. Many of us have no idea how much of goodness, strength and greatness cry within us for self-manifestation. We have mostly known only the weaker side of ourselves, which in fact belongs to the not-Self, according to Vedanta. It is the basic tragedy of our daily life that effectively prevents a real encounter with our true self. Therefore it is important for every person to know how to avoid the failure of will. The only way to do it is to cultivate the will-power.

How to generate will-power in the human system

How do we cultivate the will-power?

(a) First let us understand what exactly is will-power, in working terms. It is that positive and creative function of the mind which impels, propels and enables us to do chosen actions in a definitive way, and avoid doing unchosen actions in an equally definitive way. It is that power of the mind which enables us to do what we know to be right, and not do what we know to be wrong, under all circumstances favourable or unfavourable, known or unknown.

(b) Secondly, it is important to know and believe that will-power can be increased by everybody, without any exception, provided we are ready to apply ourselves to it and work for it steadily and methodically. Our past failures have not necessarily to be our future failures also. No one is destined to be weak all his life except him who chooses to be so. A departure for the better, nobler, higher state of existence—at least a determined effort for it—is possible at one's chosen time. It is never too early or too late to be good, true, pure and strong. Swami Vivekananda says: 'Stand up, be bold, be strong! Know that you are the creator of your own destiny. All the strength and succour you want is within yourself.'[7] What a life-giving, saving message! All the strength and succour we need is within ourselves. We should get a firm hold, an unshakable faith, in this fundamental truth.

(c) Only when we have a firm hold on this truth we can develop a will for developing the will-power. Though it may sound like a truism, it is very important to have a firm will to develop the will-power. Incredible though

---

7 *Complete Works* (1971), vol. 2, p. 225.

it may appear, many of us do not have even the will to develop the will-power! We seem to think it is big botheration, too exacting a responsibility to be carrying about all the time. But when we know for certain that within ourselves is unlimited power, that we are not these puny things as we appear to be, that we are not weak reeds worthy only to be broken anytime—then we develop the mind to manifest that power in our life, by sharply cutting out all delusions and illusions to which are the contrary.

(d) When this mind is developed, we are ready to take the most important step in developing the will-power. This step is to remove the dichotomy between the head and heart, the intellect and emotion, the thinking and feeling. How do we do it? It can be done only by loving the truth of our being. If we know it for certain that we are divine, we are the children of immortality, with a great history behind and a great destiny before, we will hate to do things which are unworthy of us, being determined to do things expected of us. In other words, our thoughts and emotions will unite in order to enable us to do the best expected of us by ourselves.

Maybe we shall not succeed without a

struggle. What of that? What is the worth of a success achieved without a struggle? We shall most certainly succeed, if we give the fight all right, without allowing hypothetical fears to sabotage our self-confidence and energy-supply.

This is the best way of fighting evil within ourselves: assert the divine and the devil will run out. How do we assert the divine within us? If we want to assert the divine, we must not do two things: we must not be cowards and we must not be hypocrites. We must be brave, take courage in both hands and follow the truth to its logical conclusion. Go with truth wherever it takes us: this should be our motto.

Opposition to this way of thinking and living will most certainly come. We must predetermine our proper attitude to such opposition and receive opposition without being overly ruffled, in good humour, with a smile, if possible. Swami Vivekananda indicates what should be our temper and attitude to oppositions. He asks:

> Have you got the will to surmount the mountain-high obstructions? If the whole world stands against you sword in hand,

WILL-POWER AND ITS DEVELOPMENT 25

would you still dare to do what you think is right? If your wives and children are against you, if all your money goes, your name dies, your wealth vanishes, would you still stick to it? Would you still pursue it and go steadily towards the goal?[8]

It is in this temper that we shall have to face opposition. You may raise the objection: to begin with, I do not have the will to surmount mountain-high obstruction. That is my problem! That is *not* your problem. Your problem is you have not adequate love for truth. Intensify the love of truth, then this temper for facing the opposition will spontaneously grow in you.

(e) Two things will oppose this creative move within us: (1) our regrets about the past, and (2) our worry about the future. Both of these are detrimental to the cultivation of will-power, because they successfully undercut all forward-looking, creative, positive movements within our minds. They are also wholly unnecessary performances. Exaggerated regrets for our past and over

---

8 *Complete Works* (1960), vol. 3, p. 226.

much worry about our future, will only damage our present, weaken our minds and injure our future also.

Now you may honestly say: how can I but regret for my past? In the past I committed many sins. Is it not my religious duty to repent for my past sins? This is an important question which requires a thorough clearing and scotching. Sloppy Vedantins are apt to make light of sin in the vain hope that their reported divinity will somehow like a sponge suck out all their bad karma, and whisk them aloft to the empyreans of *mokṣa* by a trick that is not to be explained though they continue to live indifferent lives. Vedanta acknowledges the fact of sin, but completely rejects the theory of original sin as wholly irrational. Man has nothing but original divinity and adventitious sin. Adventitious though, sin has a powerful binding effect on the soul and its free expression.

Therefore, the fact of sin has to be acknowledged as any other empirical fact. It is one thing to acknowledge the fact of sin, but it is a totally different thing to become some sort of a sin-monger, a habitual regretter. Whatever a pious face this regretting ad-infinitum may put up, psychologically it is

WILL-POWER AND ITS DEVELOPMENT

an unsound approach if you intend to get rid of it. If you are over much regretting for any sin, it is likely that you are mentally enjoying repeating the sin under the cover of righteousness.

The most important thing to be done about sin is to stop sinning, physically or mentally. How do we do it? There are a few teachings of Sri Ramakrishna which when practised will completely take care of such inner situations in the life of an earnest spiritual seeker:

> Bondage is of the mind, and freedom also is of the mind. A man is free if he constantly thinks: 'I am a free soul. How can I be bound, whether I live in the world or forest? I am a child of God, the king of kings, who can bind me?' If bitten by a snake, a man may get rid of its venom by saying emphatically, 'There is no poison in me'. In the same way, by repeating with grit and determination, 'I am not bound, I am free,' one really becomes so, one really becomes free.
>
> The wretch who constantly says, 'I am bound, I am bound' only succeeds in being bound. He who says day and night

'I am a sinner, I am a sinner,' verily becomes a sinner.

One should have such burning faith in God that one can say: 'What, I have repeated the name of God, and can sin cling to me? How can I be in bondage any more?'

If a man repeats the name of God, his body, mind and everything become pure. Why should one talk only about sin and hell, and such things? Say but once, 'O Lord, I have undoubtedly done wicked things, but I won't repeat them.' And have faith in His name.[9]

This is precisely what we have to do in regard to our past sins: Say but once in true contrition to God of your heart: 'This really I have done. Pardon me. I shall not do so again'. Then resolve to keep the word given to God. And repeat the name of God. Repetition of Lord's name will give us the power to keep our resolution

It is, however, more important that we live a wakeful life in the living present with an unencumbered free mind honestly trying to

---

9 *The Gospel* (1942), p. 138.

WILL-POWER AND ITS DEVELOPMENT   29

live according to our highest convictions. He who suffocates this moment with the worries of moments that are yet not, is doing everything possible to make his future fearful. 'In the heart of this moment is eternity!' said Meister Eckhart. And if this moment we have lived well, done our best, we may very well leave the rest. For nothing better can ever be done for future than always doing our very best right now.

We may, however, always examine our doing best and trying to find methods of even bettering our best-doing. Worry for the future is a mental disease, the medicine of which is to live entirely in this moment with all our powers poised and applied. Those who want to develop will-power must scrupulously avoid living in the past or future, and live in the living present. If we live in the present wisely according to our best light, our future cannot but be good whatever the astrologers may say.

(f) To live in the living present wisely, we require the guidance of a sound sense of values.

We should be able to persuade ourselves that we are not fooling around. We must be able to tell ourselves, in and through whatever we may be doing, that we are gradually but surely proceeding to the fulfilment of our destiny. This sound sense of values must be ascertained with due regard for our physical, mental and spiritual needs. Indian sages have ascertained such values to be four: wealth, righteousness, pleasure and liberation of the spirit.

For the generality of mankind, physical and emotional starvation is not conducive to the cultivation of will-power or development of higher life. As starvation is bad, surfeit is also disastrous. For the fulfilment of our physical and emotional needs, we require wealth. But if we earn wealth unrighteously, we release some forces which will eventually jump upon us like tigers and that will not be good for our will-power at all. Hence, both the values of pleasure and wealth have to be obedient to the laws of righteousness or *dharma*. But this righteousness, again, shall be inspired by a higher motive which is the attainment of the liberation of the spirit.

When we function in our daily life in accordance with this sound sense of values, we stay protected within a fire-ring of wisdom, as it were, which the evils of life cannot easily penetrate. Then we live in the

WILL-POWER AND ITS DEVELOPMENT

forceful conviction of living rightly without a trace of guilt sense. It is this guilt sense with or without reason that eats away the roots of will-power. When we live not only without a guilt sense, but positively with a sense of living rightly, we get hold of a power of conviction which releases a new force within us. And this force immensely helps the development of will-power.

Cultivate one power of conviction at least, if you want to develop the will-power. Believe with your whole soul you are on the right path; do not doubt everything all the time. This is not intelligence. Believe in Vedanta, in Ramakrishna, or in your own Atman, with all your might, and you will see how the will-power grows as if from nowhere. One thing rightly and powerfully done somewhere within oneself will help doing other things also.

(g) Now, this sound sense of values requires to be zealously guarded, for we are being constantly assailed by chaotic winds of various contrary ideas.

How do we guard the sense of value? We can do so by doing three things: (i) by constant discrimination between the real and the unreal; (ii) by keeping ourselves busy doing those things that we have decidedly accepted as beneficial; and (iii) by avoiding idle curiosity about things which do not concern our main pursuit in life.

What through proper scrutiny and discrimination we decided to be beneficial, we must just force ourselves to do, if necessary by putting our own knee on our own chest, and boldly face the consequence. The hardest task in the world is not 'bringing up father' or bringing up children, but bringing up oneself! To one who knows how to discipline oneself, his other tasks will become easy. There is a case for doing some sort of a careful rough-handling of oneself, in order to break down the barriers which impede the flow of the will-power. 'Do the right thing right now,' should be our day's order to the mind. That should be the principle. Instead of doing the wrong things hurriedly and repenting at leisure, is it not better to do the right thing promptly and enjoy the blessings of such actions at leisure?

If we ourselves are unable to decide what is right or wrong, counsel should be sought from the teacher. If the teacher is not available, guidance may be taken from scriptures. But even when we have decided upon a right

WILL-POWER AND ITS DEVELOPMENT

action, many considerations will try to oppose its prompt execution. 'All are acting differently': will be one plea. Then there will be considerations of what they call 'worldly wisdom'. Much of the 'worldly wisdom' stuff is but a rationalization of our weaknesses compounded with the idea of what is supposed to be self-interest. And these considerations will be manipulated by our own mind. We have to carefully discern here the attempted sabotage of our good efforts to develop the will-power by the unregenerate or wicked part of our mind. We should then firmly slash down this opposition by that part of the mind which has already allied itself with truth. On the other hand, what we have known to be definitely wrong and harmful, we must as promptly stop doing that and boldly face the consequences.

Thoughtless people may ridicule us for standing apart, selfish people may torment us for not doing wrong things, even our friends may regard our behaviour as strange. Yet we must follow what we have realized to be true and right. However, we must be extremely cautious, circumspect and also deep-seeing in ascertaining what is right, and what is wrong. We must not impulsively jump into conclusions and then move ahead in a fanatical manner. That will harm the development of will-power. If, left to ourselves, we are unable to determine what is right and what is wrong, we should take the help of those who know the answer, and then act upon what we have learnt.

On the basis of whatever we have thus learnt and determined, we should ourselves plan a simple routine for our daily life. This routine should be planned keeping in view that we are seeking daily self-preservation and self-improvement on all levels, physical, mental and spiritual. It should be so planned that our human relations, recreational needs, ideals and aspirations—everything could be actualized through that routine. No matter what happens, we should then follow that routine. In the preliminary stage this is a very helpful method to get a firm grip on the mind. Our senses will have to obey our decisions made with due circumspection.

Exceptional cases may arise when the routine will have to be set aside—as for instance, when there is serious accident in the house, or a friend has died—but as soon as possible we should again return to our routine. At a later stage when we have made up sufficient leeway by succeeding in controlling the vagaries of our mind, we may adjust the routine according to the higher needs of our self-development.

(h) It is extremely important to remember that in developing will-power the greatest help will come from the power of concentration we have already attained. In fact these two always go together. The power of concentration helps the growth and development of will-power, and will-power helps the power of concentration.

How can we increase the power of concentration? The simplest way to do it is to pour our whole mind into the work on hand, whether it is cooking, polishing shoes, playing basket ball, watching birds, experimenting in the laboratory or praying in the chapel. In other words, when you are meditating, you must not be seeing the movie!

(i) And for this we require a sufficient reserve of mental energy. That is to say, in order to develop the will-power we must stop all squandering of our mental energy. This squandering of mental energy is done through useless talks, purposeless work, futile controversies, wild fantasies, backbiting, day-dreaming, lewd thinking, concern for things which is none of one's business, hypothetical fears and finding fault with others. To build up a sufficient storage of mental energy, which is so necessary for motoring the will-power, we must stop doing things which drain our mental energy.

We will notice that men of powerful will are men of few words. People always wait to attentively listen to what they have to say. They are not pining to be interesting or exciting. They live with a purpose, for an ideal. They are immensely dynamic, but they are poised, intense but not tense. They are not easily shaken by anything.

(j) The conservation of mental energy in its turn will depend on the conservation of physical energy especially sex energy. Those who thoughtlessly or deliberately squander their physical energy are bound to have shallow minds. And shallow minds have poor will-power. Therefore in the educational system of ancient India supreme importance was attached to the practice of *brahmacarya*, continence, so much so that the period of studentship itself was called *brahmacarya*. The main secret of developing will-power lies in the proper practice of *brahmacarya*. Therefore, for developing the will-power we must conserve our physical energy. Physical energy is conserved by living a moral life of purity and moderation. In moderation is suppleness; in suppleness is strength.

(k) Lastly, to develop the will-power we must never take our failures seriously. We must not lose heart in the face of repeated failures. For there is no other way to success except through repeated failures. Failures should be accepted as a part of the whole game, as steps to mount the pedestal of success. These steps when followed rightly, will surely help us in developing the will-power.

'Goodness gracious,' some of us are apt to think, 'if it takes all that for developing the will-power, let the Swamis have them all, we better go for a snack!' Well, this is not all, there is more to it. Snacks have a place in life. But it may not be forgotten that will-power has no substitute whatsoever. We cannot get any worthy thing without paying for it.

Remedies for failure of will-power

A situation may, however, arise when we discover that after doing all these to the best of our supposed ability, our will-power is not yet sufficiently strong. What should we do in such a situation? We should stop, think and analyse the whole situation. And we will most certainly discover that the failure of the will is taking place in a subtle way through a wrong thought process. It is thought that gets translated into action. If the thought is wrong how can the action be right? Therefore to strengthen the will-power to the expected degree we should work on the thought process.

How to work on the thought process, or control thought? This by itself is a major subject for discussion. For our present purpose it will be sufficient to know that 'working on the thought process' here means prevention of wrong movements of thought.

In one sermon Buddha specially instructs on thought control. In the conclusion of that sermon, summarizing his precepts, the Buddha said:

Remember, Bhikkhus, the only way to become victorious over wrong thoughts is to review from time to time the phases of one's mind, to reflect over them, to root out all that is evil, and cultivate all that is good.

When at last a Bhikku has become victorious over his wrong thoughts...he becomes the master of his mind, conquering desire and thus ending evil for all time.[10]

One who has become victorious over wrong thoughts cannot but have that will-power which will never fail. Now, when we proceed to practise the precept, '...root out all that is evil and cultivate all that is good,' we find that it is something more than what we can do. What should we do when we discover our utter inner helplessness and shameful weakness? If we realize our true weakness, we should then humbly do the easiest thing. We should pray to God for will-power. It is an infallible method.

There are problems of both fulfilled and unfulfilled prayer. But in regard to the prayer for will-power we have a definite imperative of Sri Ramakrishna. Among the few things Sri Ramakrishna has definitively asked us to pray

---

10 Sudhakar Dikshit, *Sermons and Sayings of the Buddha*, pp. 42–43.

to God for, will-power is one. His precept in this regard is that we should earnestly pray to God for will-power, so that we may be able to do what is right, and desist from doing what is wrong, so that we may be able to devote ourselves to the practice of spiritual disciplines. Moreover he has asked us—and this is very important—to also pray that our entire will with all its power may be united with God's will.

Caution needed for properly directing will-power

There is, however, one important point to be noted in the development of will-power: the will must be given a right direction. All the notorious evil geniuses in history who inflicted on humanity unspeakable suffering, such as Hitler and his tribe, also had a kind of powerful will. That kind of will-power can only create bondage for oneself and miseries for others. We are not trying to develop that kind of malevolent will-power. But we are trying to develop the benign will-power from which no evil can ever come, but only good. The perfection of such will-power is attained only when one is able to say with all joy and spontaneity: 'Lord, Thy will be done, not my will!'

At a certain stage when the will-power is taking shape, great care and caution should be taken to direct it entirely to God. And this is done through prayer as taught by Sri Ramakrishna. What could be a simpler method of developing the will-power than prayer? Along with prayer, ideally goes repetition of Lord's name. Many Indian mystics and saints are unanimous in their teachings that, spiritually speaking, there is nothing we cannot attain by mere loving repetition of Lord's name. Who is there so weak, so unfortunate as cannot even take the Lord's name?

In any case, whether we are weak or strong, prayer and repetition of Lord's name will always help us in developing will-power, for these two practices remove all evil thoughts and purify our mind. We must take all care to hunt out all our inner blemishes from their hide-outs and acknowledge them to ourselves and to God within us. We will gain a whole world of strength by doing so.

But we must not go about speaking about our weaknesses to all and sundry. That way no one is helped. We should, however, without reservation, speak about them, in case of need, only to our personal teachers and to no one else. Be sure there are many unscrupulous people in the world who will take every advantage of your uncalled for confessions. Consciousness of our utter helplessness leads us to self-surrender. Self-surrender, when true and complete, shatters all our inner bondages which cause failure of our will. Then suddenly the prostrate-person springs up as the very picture of inner power. No one understands whence has come so much power within him. Says Jesus Christ, 'Without Me Ye can do nothing.' How true! Without God's grace we can do nothing. In other words, with God's grace we can do everything.

When we practise prayer, meditation, repetition of Lord's name, God is already with us. And this fact expresses itself as the purity of mind. This is becoming strong in God's strength. It is the will of the pure mind that is invincible. Through the help of such a will one can attain even the highest, which is God.

Behold the triumph of will-power

The most magnificent story of the

triumph of will-power is that of a man who did not ask from God a thing, who did not even acknowledge God. He is Buddha. And this proves the potency of the human will per se. It is inspiring to know this.

You all know the story of his life. After renouncing the world, his home, throne, wife, a newly born son and all, Siddhartha became a monk. Then he went in search of a teacher. He studied under several teachers, learnt from them whatever they had to teach, but was not satisfied with anyone's teaching. All the teachers loved and respected him. But Siddhartha, not yet Buddha, stayed dissatisfied. He now realized that all these classical teachers had not the answer for his search which was to find a way out for the cessation of *duḥkha* or miseries inherent in human life. So he decided to blaze his own path. Alone, homeless, this leonine seeker of truth came to Rajagriha and began to stay in Ratnagiri. There he became acquainted with king Bimbisara (who, after Siddhartha's enlightenment, became his disciple). It was at Bimbisara's court that Siddhartha offered his life in exchange of that of a lamb which was going to be sacrified. From Ratnagiri for the convenience of quiet practice of spiritual disciplines he came to Uruvela, which is now known as the famous Buddha-Gaya. At Uruvela, for six long years Siddhartha practised frightful austerities and reduced his golden body into skin and bone, his resolution being: either I realize the truth or the body falls.

One day when, after bathing in the river Niranjana, he was returning to his cottage, he fell down out of sheer exhaustion! He was taken for dead. But he regained consciousness. Then Siddhartha realized this was not the path to enlightenment, this extreme austerity. One village maiden who had come to worship gave him rice-milk and he accepted the gift. When he had partaken of the rice-milk all his limbs were refreshed, his mind became clear again and he was strong to receive the highest enlightenment. As he reduced his austerities, firmer became his resolution for realization. Then on one full-moon night of the month of Vaisakha, he took his seat under the now famous Bo-tree with this resolution: 'Let my body dry out on this seat, let my skin, bone and flesh wither away, but before attaining illumination which is rarely ever found even in many ages, I am not going to move from this seat.'[11]

The rest of the story may be narrated in the words of Ashvaghosha's Life of the Buddha. Expressed in the language of legends though, the narration brings home the triumph of the will-power with a marvellous impact on human civilization itself. It is said:

> The Holy One directed his steps to that blessed Bodhi-tree beneath whose shade he should accomplish his search.
> As he walked, the earth shook, and a brilliant light transfigured the world.
> When he sat down, the heavens resounded with joy, and all living beings were filled with good cheer.
> Mara (the evil spirit) alone, lord of the five desires, bringer of death and enemy of truth, was grieved and rejoiced not. With his three daughters, the tempters, and with his host of evil demons, he went to

---

11 इहासने शुष्यतु मे शरीरं
त्वगस्थिमांसं प्रलयञ्च यातु ।
अप्राप्य बोधिं बहुकल्पदुर्लभां
नैवासनात् कायमेतश्चलिष्यते ॥

the place where the great *shramana* sat. But Sakyamuni minded him not. Mara uttered fear-inspiring threats and raised a whirl-storm so that the skies were darkened and the ocean roared and trembled. But the Blessed One under the Bodhi-tree remained calm and feared not. The Enlightened One knew that no harm could befall him.

The three daughters of Mara tempted Bodhisattva but he paid no attention to them and when Mara saw that he could kindle no desire in the heart of the victorious *Shramana*, he ordered all evil spirits at his command to attack him and over awe the great *muni*.

But the Blessed One watched them as one would watch harmless games of children. All the fierce hatred of the evil spirit was of no avail. The flames of hell became wholesome breezes of perfume, and the angry thunderbolts were changed into lotus blossoms.

When the Mara saw this, he fled away with his army from the Bodhi-tree. Whilst from above a rain of heavenly flowers fell, and voices of good spirits were heard:

Blessed the great *muni*! his mind unmoved by hatred; the host of the wicked one has not over-awed him. He is pure and wise, loving and full of mercy.
As the rays of the sun drowns the darkness of the world, so he who perseveres in his search, will find the truth, and the truth will enlighten him.[12]

Siddhartha having thus put to flight Mara, gave himself up to meditation. And that very night seated on the same seat, he attained illumination and became Tathagata, the Buddha. Such is the magnificent story of the world's greatest triumph of human will-power.

The great option open to all

None of us is absolutely devoid of will-power. Otherwise, we could not have been what we are right now. But it remains a fact, that whatever may be the varying

---

[12] Paul Carus, *The Gospel of Buddha* (New York: The Open Court Publishing House Company, 1921), pp. 38–39

qualities of our already attained degrees of will-power, the more the will-power directed Godward, the nobler human beings we shall become. And those adventurous souls who will not stay content being noble human beings, will realize the Truth, extending further their will-power.

By God's grace so much always stays open to man. How much are we going to take?